CONTENT

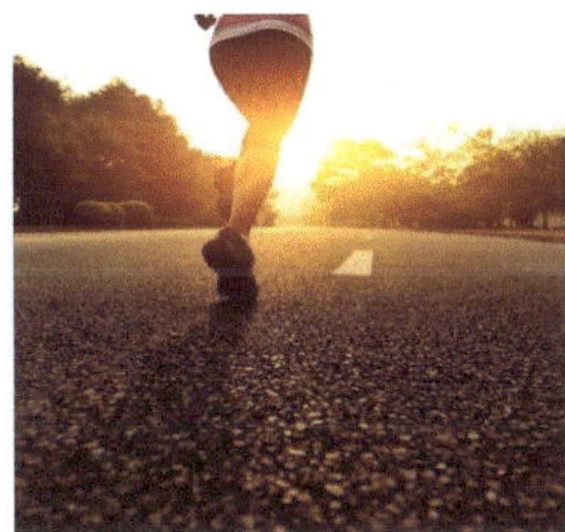
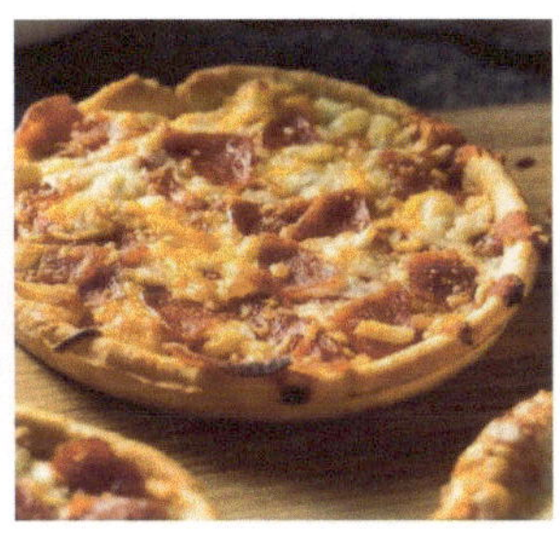
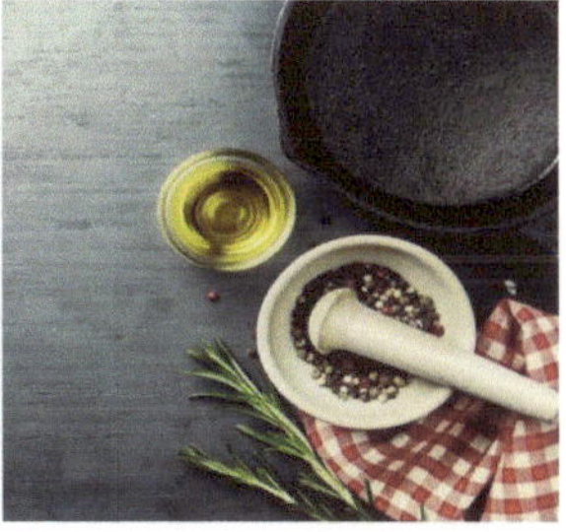

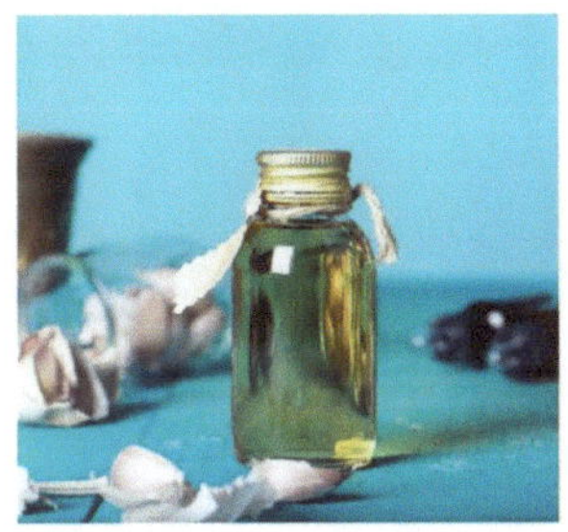
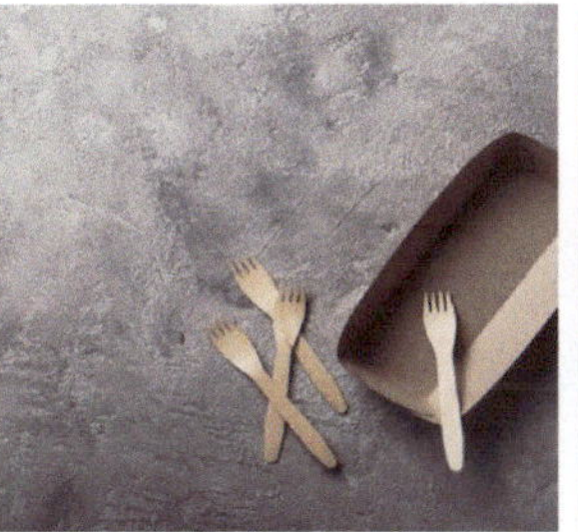
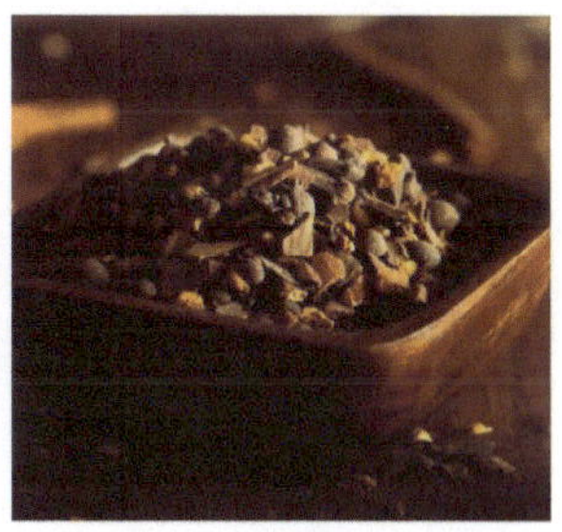

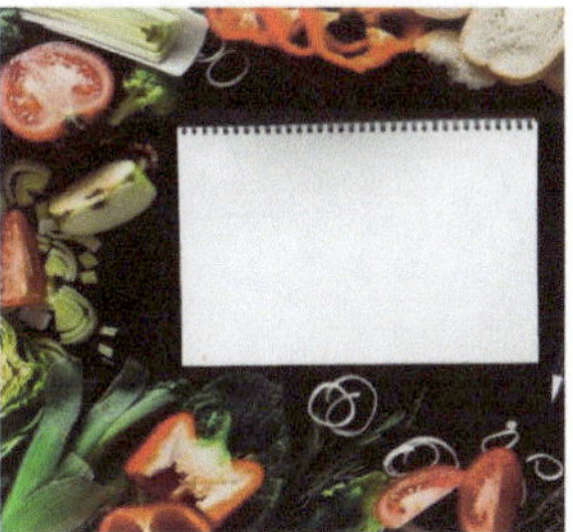

Disclaimer

- ➢ This book is written with the intention to create awareness
- ➢ You choose to use these instructions with your own discretions
- ➢ This is not a replacement of your current medication – You have to continue using your medicine and this process will help you to get better over time
- ➢ If you have any allergy please consult your doctor before consuming any of these foods
- ➢ If you have any serious illness please consult your doctor before consuming any of these foods

PREFACE

Let's understand the basics of human body:

- ➢ Human body is made up of cells
- ➢ Digestive system is the engine of human body
- ➢ The food we eat is broken down into nutrients. Nutrients are then absorbed across the gut valve into blood
- ➢ Then your circulatory system including your blood carry the nutrients from the food you break down and the oxygen you breath to the cells of human body
- ➢ So, if the right nutrients are reaching to our cells, our cells have right raw material to do all of the functions to help you in preventing your body from diseases and help you to recover from the existing diseases
- ➢ Your skin, hair, weight everything is controlled by what your cells get
- ➢ If you feed your cells junk your cells don't get what they require and you will soon feel hungry until the cells get the desired nutrients
- ➢ These cells need energy to function. Without energy these cells die and that is where every disease starts from
  - o Say no to dieting
  - o Eat right food – both quality and quantity
- ➢ When you follow a natural cycle, you don't have to diet. Just follow the rhythm of human body
- ➢ It's your body and no one knows about it better than you. You have to believe that your body can heal
- ➢ Human body is interconnected. So, we just can't treat it without treating the root cause
  - o For example – high blood pressure can flush more calcium out of your body which ultimately can lead to osteoporosis
  - o So here the root cause is not calcium deficiency but high blood pressure and you have to address high blood pressure here to prevent osteoporosis

Through this book we will discuss the lifestyle and dietary changes which will address all such root causes.

We will then learn about certain healthy and tasty recipes which we can include in our meals.

Step 1 – Lifestyle Changes

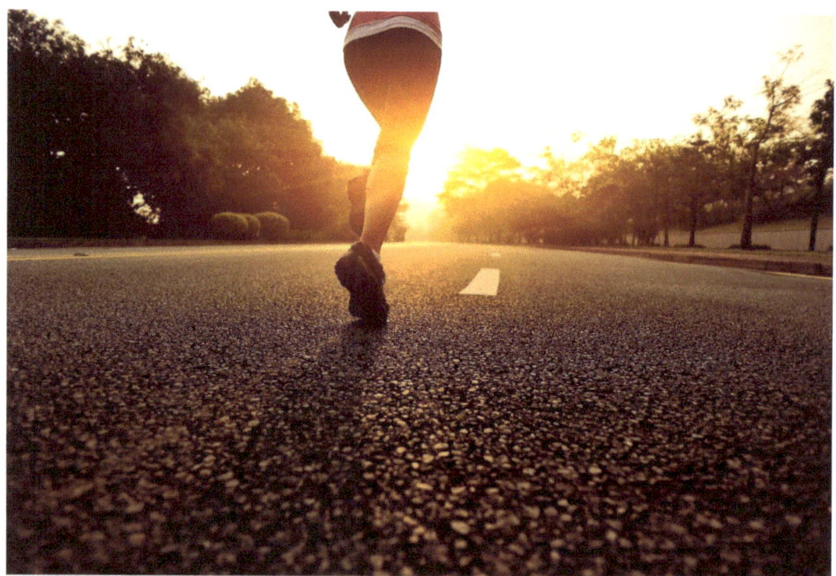

- ➢ Sleep
    - o At least 6-7 hours of sound sleep
    - o Sleep at around same time daily and similarly wake up at same time

- ➢ Emotional Health
    - o Everyone has problems; it is how you face it. Keep calm
    - o Deep breathing for 5 minutes
        - ▪ Slow inhale and slow exhale
        - ▪ 1.5 hours before every meal and just before sleep

- ➢ Self-Discipline
    - o Walk 30 minutes per day
    - o Yoga/Exercise for at least 15 minutes per day
    - o There will be parties, weddings and festivals. Enjoy those but you have to keep yourself on track. Have a blast and get back to life of discipline
    - o Even if you want to socialize daily just remember a golden rule –
        - ▪ SOCIALIZING IS NOT EATING
    - o Eat the food at home and socialize. Get along with your friends and family; have a good time, share your experience, have laugh but try to limit outside food
    - o Don't remove it entirely from your life just limit it to once a week to start with and maybe reduce it to twice a month afterwards

Step 2 – Dietary Changes

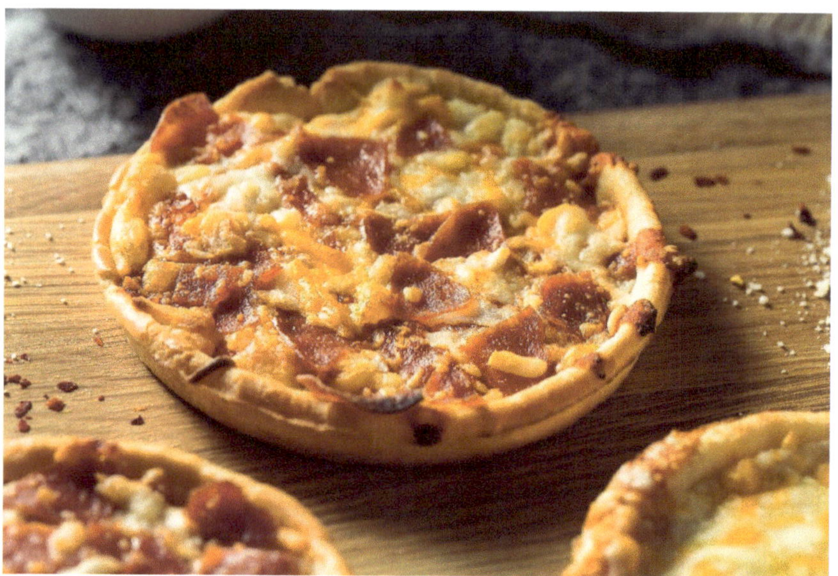

- ➢ Stop eating junk and processed foods
- ➢ Don't reuse cooking oil
- ➢ Don't miss your meal
- ➢ Eat slowly
- ➢ Coffee/Tea – Limit to 1 cup/day
- ➢ Refined sugar and refined oil – Out of life
- ➢ Limit alcohol
  - o Limit it once a week first and then to twice a month
  - o Don't over drink in a single sitting
- ➢ Early dinner
  - o Gap of at least 3 hours between dinner and bed time
  - o Excuses –
    - ▪ Come home late –Carry your dinner
    - ▪ Work late – have dinner and work
    - ▪ Social life – Remember the golden rule: Socializing is not eating
- ➢ Water
  - o Don't drink with meals
  - o Wait for at least 30 minutes after any meal
  - o Sit down and drink
  - o Don't drink too quickly, sip it slowly

Step 3 – Dietary Inclusions

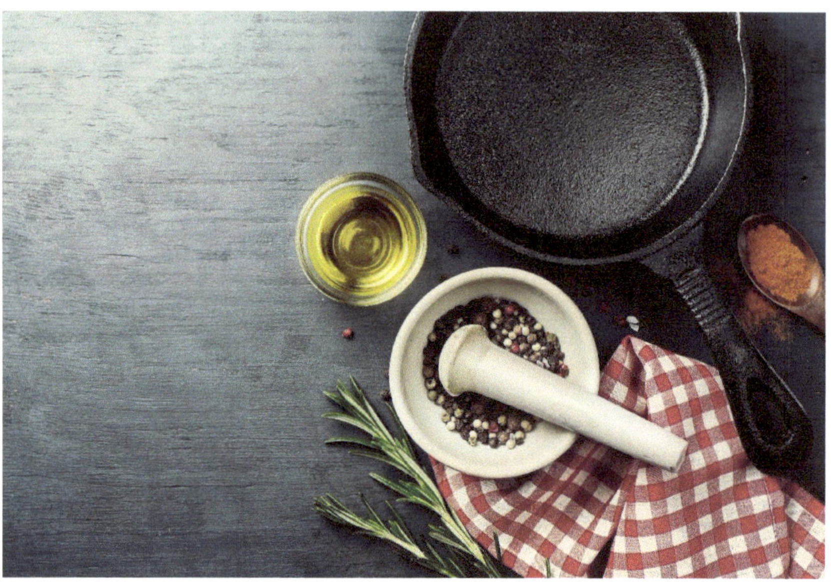

- ➢ 2 glass warm water
    - o Drink slowly just after you wake up
- ➢ Turmeric, black pepper, pure ghee/virgin cold pressed coconut oil
    - o 1/2 teaspoon turmeric, ¼ teaspoon black pepper and 1 teaspoon pure ghee or cold pressed virgin coconut oil
    - o Mix well and eat empty stomach – at least 30 minutes before breakfast
    - o Don't take if you are suffering with any kidney disease
- ➢ Curd, Garlic and onions
    - o 1 bowl curd or yogurt with lunch
    - o ½ onion and 2-3 cloves raw garlic with dinner
- ➢ 1 Cardamom, 1 teaspoon Fennel seeds, small piece of chemical free jaggery just after lunch and dinner
- ➢ ½ teaspoon Indian Gooseberry (Amla) powder 1 hour after lunch with warm water
- ➢ Sweet potato
    - o Boil and spray salt and lemon as per taste
    - o Eat as evening snack 2-3 times a week
- ➢ Lemon grass
    - o Grow it in your lawn/pot or buy dry powder online
    - o Add ½ teaspoon in your tea or in boiling water
    - o Once a day, 1 hour after dinner
    - o Don't take if you are suffering with any kidney disease

Step 4 – Oil Pulling

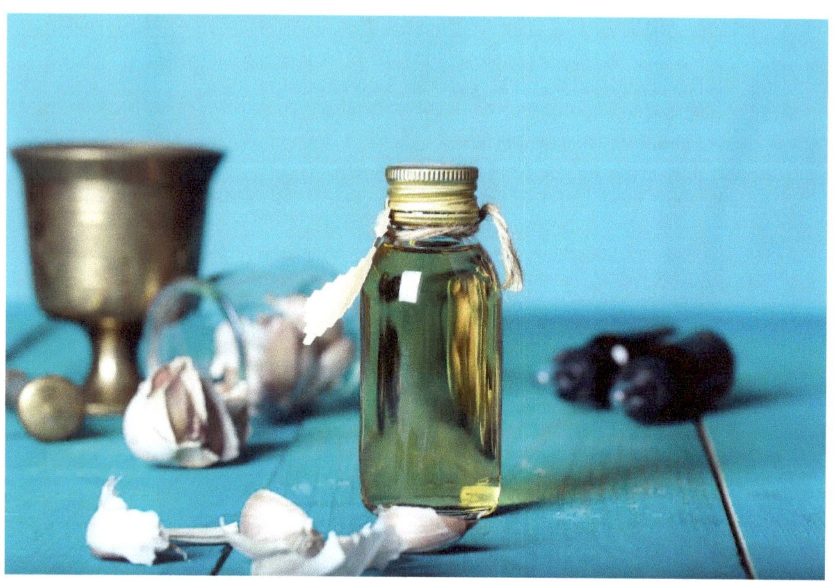

Oral health, Overall health!!

- There is a relationship between **oral health** and **overall** wellness. Gum disease is linked to a lot of illnesses including heart disease, diabetes, respiratory disease, osteoporosis, and rheumatoid arthritis
- Oil pulling is an ancient remedy to whiten your teeth, freshen your breath and greatly improve your oral health
- Put a tablespoon of extra-virgin coconut oil in your mouth, swish it around for 15–20 minutes
- Do it just after or before brushing your teeth as per your comfort
- It reduces the number of harmful bacteria in the mouth

Step 5 – Intermittent Fasting

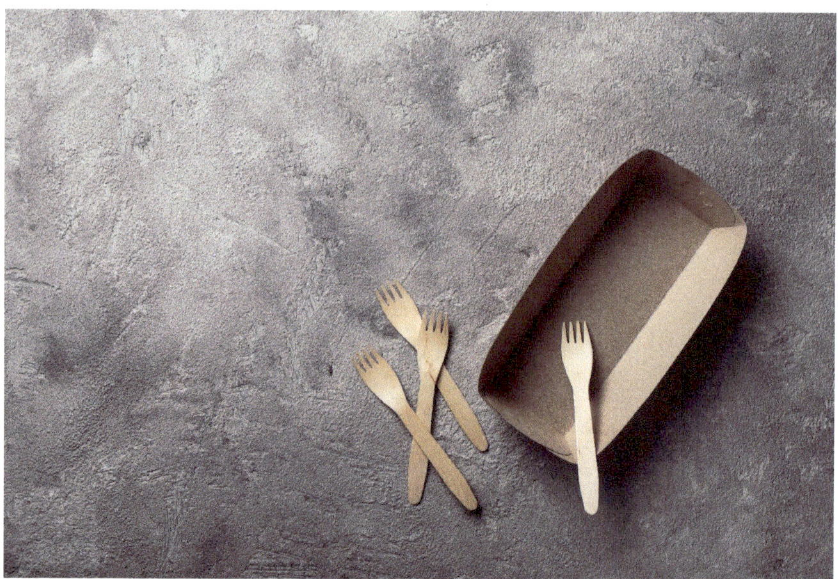

Intermittent fasting – 2 times a week

> 16:8 intermittent fasting is a form of time-restricted fasting. It involves consuming foods during an 8-hour window and avoiding food, or fasting, for the remaining 16 hours
> The easiest way to follow the 16:8 diet is to choose a 16-hour fasting window that includes the time that a person spends sleeping
> It is advisable to finish food consumption in the early evening, as metabolism slows down after this time
> People may choose one of the following 8-hour eating windows:
>   o 9 a.m. to 5 p.m.
>   o 10 a.m. to 6 p.m.
>   o Noon to 8 p.m.

Some people may need to experiment to find the best eating window and mealtimes for their lifestyle.

Step 6 – Garam Masala

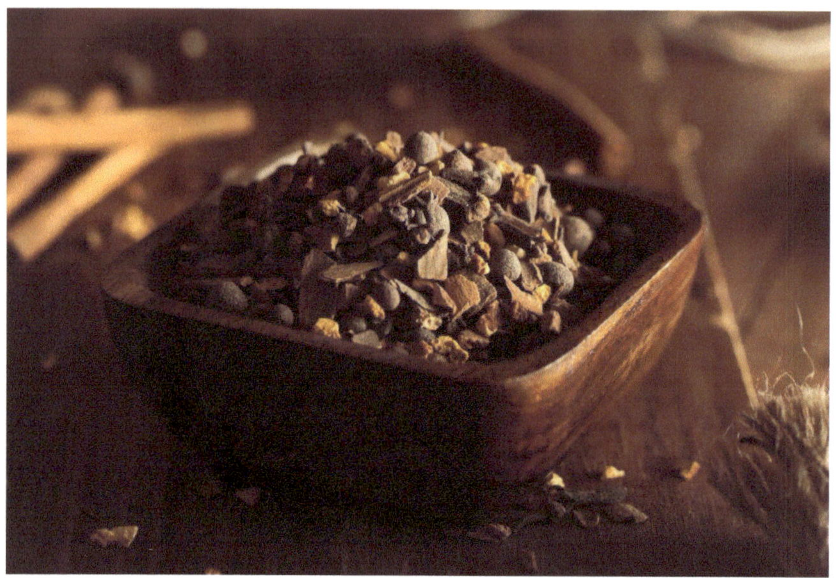

A simple homemade powder made from specific spices that help to boost our immunity. We need to include this masala in every dish/curry we consume on daily basis.

- Taste enhancer
- Immunity booster
- Perfect for cold & flu season
- Safe for kids

Ingredients:

- 7 tbsp. – Turmeric powder
- 4 tbsp – Cumin seeds
- 4 tbsp – Coriander Seeds
- 7 tbsp- Fennel seeds
- 2 tbsp- Dry Ginger Powder
- 2 tbsp – Whole black pepper
- 1/2 tbsp – Sri Lankan Rolled Cinnamon powder
- 3 tbsp – Cardamom powder

Method:

1. Keep turmeric powder and dry ginger powder in a separate bowl (no roasting)
2. Lightly roast all the remaining ingredients on a slow flame till you get a nice aroma (avoid burning of spices)
3. Let the mixture cool, transfer that in a grinder and grind to make a fine powder.
4. Add turmeric and dry ginger powder to it and mix with a dry spoon.
5. Store in a clean, air tight jar

How to consume?

- ½ teaspoon per person
- Can be consumed everyday
- Use it as an alternative of your spices while making curry or use it as a seasoning

Who can consume?

- Everyone in the family to improve the immunity (anyone having allergies or any specific disease, please consult your doctor before consuming)
- Great for kids to elderly people of a family

Step 7 – Healthy Recipes

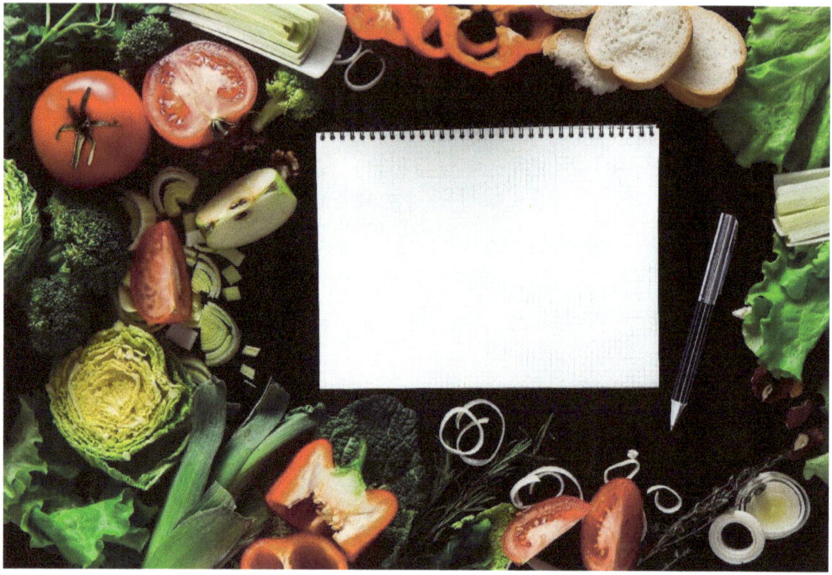

Below recipes are just a way to show how you can bring a change by following these methods of cooking. You can cook any recipe of your choice by taking these methods into consideration. Preparing healthy food is the ultimate objective here.

Sprouts Salad

Ingredients:

- 2 cups of sprouted moong beans
- 1 small or medium sized cucumber chopped
- 1 medium sized tomato, finely chopped
- 1 green chili
- 1/4 tsp garam masala (optional)
- 1 tsp lemon juice or as required
- 1 boiled sweet potato
- A few coriander leaves for garnishing
- Rock salt or black salt as per taste

Method:

- Rinse the sprouted moong beans in water
- Boil them till they are completely cooked
- Strain the cooked sprouts
- Mix all the ingredients except the salt and lemon juice in a bowl
- Season with salt and add a few drops of lemon juice
- Garnish with coriander leaves
- Should be consumed immediately

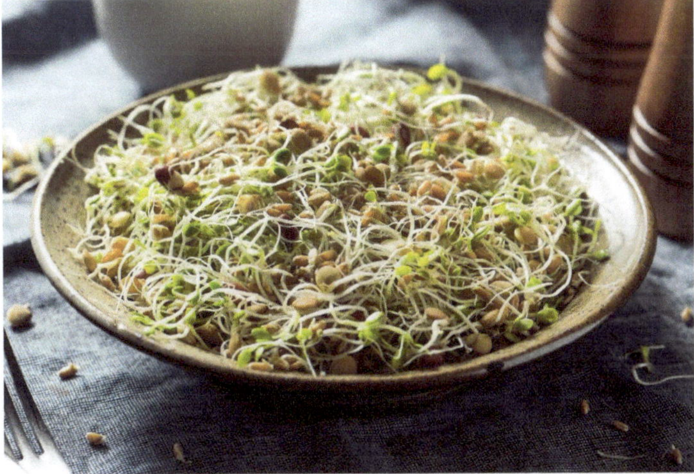

Mango Salad

Ingredients:

- 1 ripe mango, diced
- ½ medium red bell pepper, chopped
- ¼ cup chopped onion
- ¼ cup packed fresh cilantro or parsley leaves, chopped
- 1 jalapeño, seeded and minced
- ¼ cup lime juice
- Rock Salt to taste

Method:

1. In a serving bowl, mix mango, bell pepper, onion, cilantro/parsley and jalapeño
2. Drizzle the lime juice and mix well
3. Add salt as per taste
4. Keep the mixture for 10 minutes for a better taste

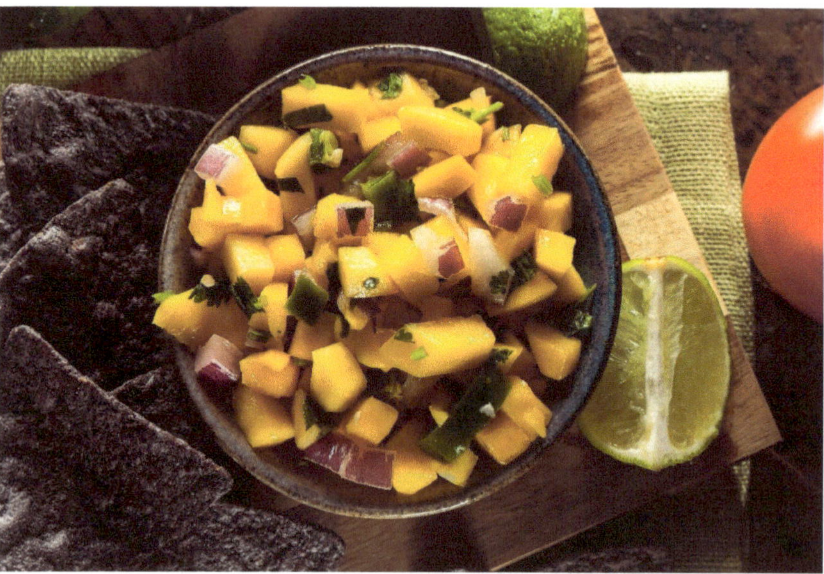

Sprouts Roll

Ingredients:

- 1 cup sprouted and steamed mung
- ½ cup yogurt or 1 tbsp lemon juice
- 1 cup cilantro
- 1 green chili, small piece of ginger and 3-5 cloves garlic
- 1 tbsp sesame seeds
- 1 tbsp jaggery
- 1 tsp coriander and cumin powder
- ½ tsp turmeric powder
- 2 cups whole wheat flour
- Pure ghee
- Salt to taste

Method:

1. Add curd, sprouted moong, ginger, garlic and chili in a blender. Make a smooth paste
2. In a mixing bowl add all spice ingredients, moong paste, salt, jaggery, sesame seeds and 2 tablespoons of ghee. Mix thoroughly.
3. Add flour and knead it into a smooth soft dough. Cover it and keep aside for at least 10 minutes.
4. Roll the dough balls and keep it a little bit thicker than chapati
5. Roast it nicely on both sides by applying ghee
6. Consume immediately

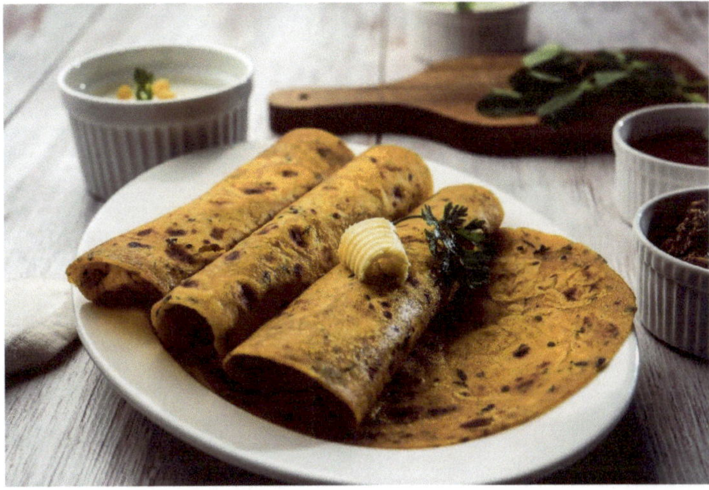

Sattu Pancake

Ingredients:

- 1 cup sattu flour
- 1/4 tsp cinnamon
- 1/4 tsp salt
- 1 tbsp jaggery powder
- 1 banana
- 1 tbsp pure ghee
- 3/4 cup coconut milk
- Chopped nuts for garnishing

Method:

1. Sift the flour into the mixing bowl and add jaggery powder, salt and cinnamon. Mix together.
2. Mash the banana in a bowl, add ghee and coconut milk. Mix with a ladle to get it to batter consistency.
3. Heat the pan, add ghee. Add the batter, flip it and cook until its browned from both sides.
4. Garnish with chopped nuts and serve hot

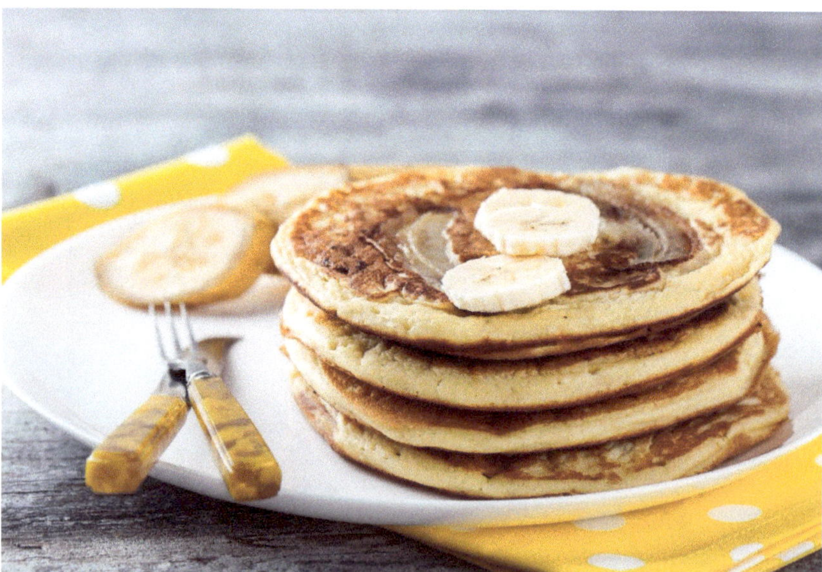

Cucumber Banana Smoothie

Ingredients:

- 1 cucumber
- 1 banana
- ½ lemon
- Small piece of ginger
- Small pinch of black pepper
- ½ teaspoon of cumin powder
- A few fresh leaves of coriander
- A few fresh leaves of mint
- Rock salt or black salt as per taste

Method:

- Put all the things into a mixer grinder
- Add some water
- Blend it very fine
- Add more water as per consistency requirement
- You may add some ice cubes in summers
- Should be consumed immediately

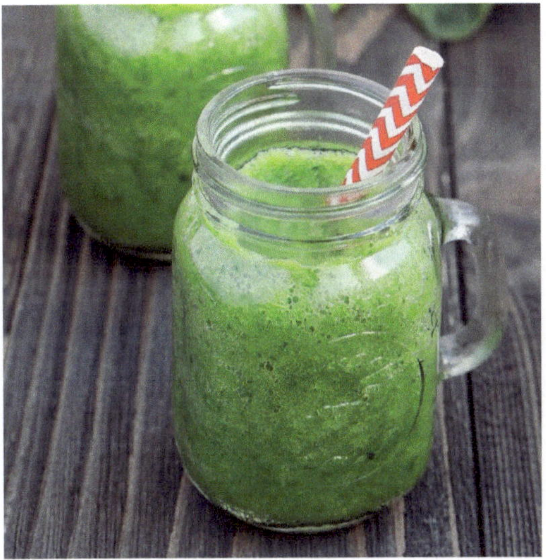

Oats Smoothie

Ingredients:

- 2 tablespoons oats
- 1 cup curd
- 1 small green chili
- Small pinch of black pepper
- ½ teaspoon of cumin powder
- A few fresh leaves of coriander
- A few fresh leaves of mint
- Rock salt or black salt as per taste

Method:

- Wash the oats thoroughly under running water
- Boil with some water and then filter it
- Let it cool
- Blend the curd
- Grind fresh mint leaves and add it to curd with a pinch of black pepper and black salt
- Mix the oats and blend all the things properly
- Should be consumed immediately

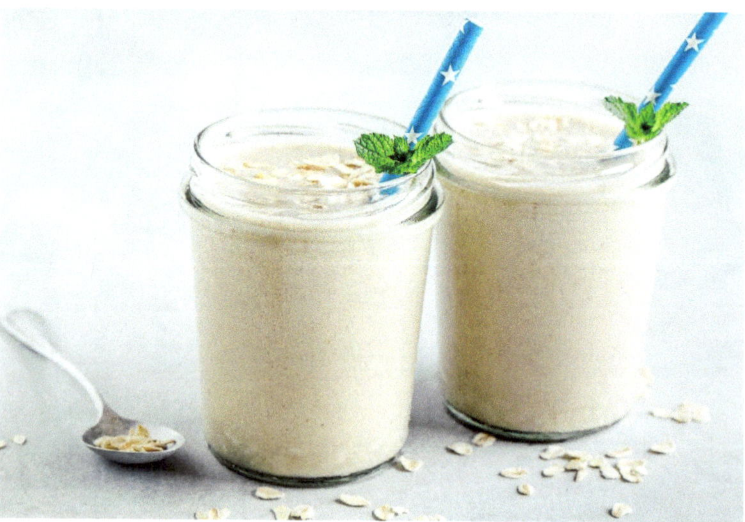

Spinach Smoothie

Ingredients:

- ½ cup of fresh spinach leaves
- ½ teaspoon lemon juice
- 1 teaspoon honey
- Small pinch of black pepper
- ½ teaspoon of cumin powder
- Rock salt or black salt as per taste

Method:

- Mix spinach leaves, cumin powder, honey, lemon juice, black pepper and black salt
- Grind it with half glass of water
- Blend the mixture very fine
- Should be consumed immediately
- You may add some ice cubes in summers

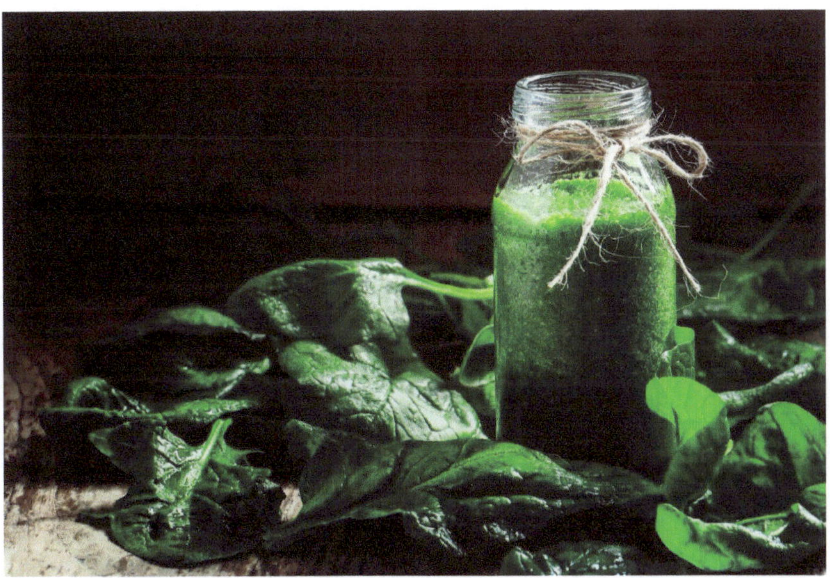

Carrot, Beetroot and Apple Smoothie

Ingredients:

- 2 carrots
- ½ beetroot
- 1 apple
- 1 teaspoon honey
- ½ teaspoon lemon juice
- Small pinch of black pepper
- ½ teaspoon of cumin powder
- Rock salt or black salt as per taste

Method:

- Cut carrot, beetroot and apple into small pieces
- Mix those with cumin powder, honey, lemon juice, black pepper and black salt
- Grind the mixture with half glass of water
- Blend the mixture very fine
- Should be consumed immediately
- You may add some ice cubes in summers

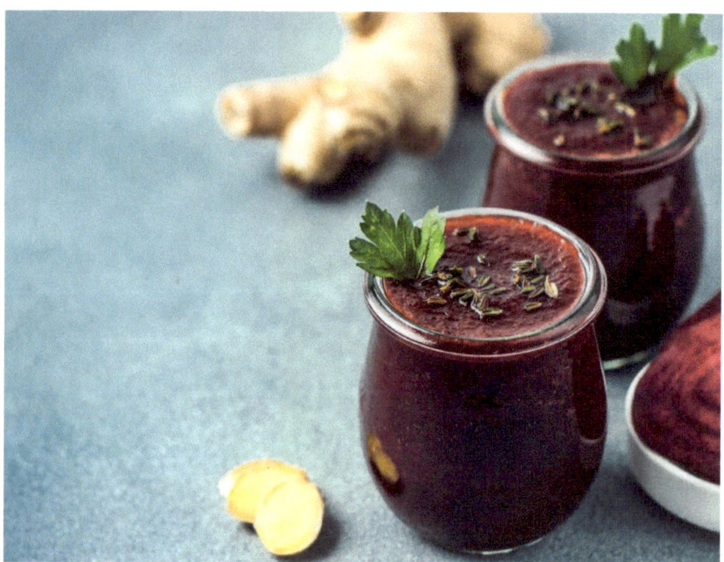

Mix Fruit Smoothie

Ingredients:

- 1 kiwi fruit
- A handful of grapes
- 1 apple
- 1 teaspoon honey
- ½ teaspoon lemon juice
- Some mint leaves
- A little piece of ginger
- Small pinch of black pepper
- Rock salt or black salt as per taste

Method:

- Cut kiwi fruit and apple into small pieces
- Mix those with grapes, mint leaves, honey, lemon juice, black pepper, ginger and black salt
- Grind the mixture with half glass of water
- Blend the mixture very fine
- Should be consumed immediately
- You may add some ice cubes in summers

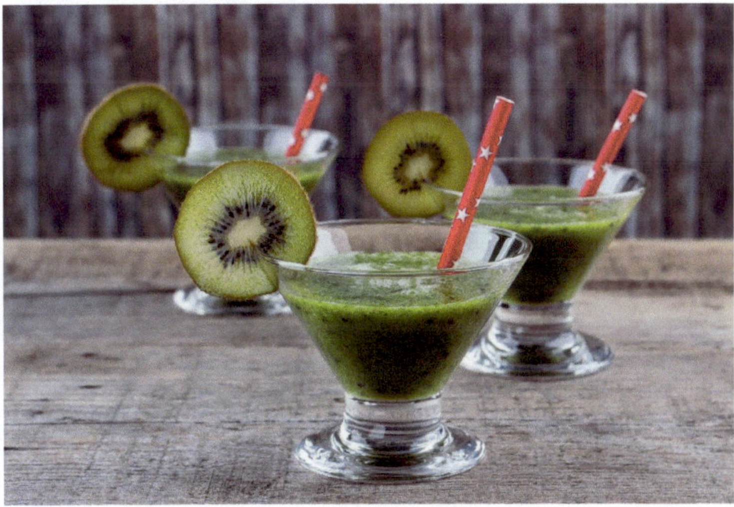

Green Tea

Ingredients:

- 1 tbsp green tea
- ¼ tsp oregano
- 1 tsp fennel
- ½ tsp carom
- Pinch of pepper
- 2-3 sprigs thyme
- 1-2 sprigs rosemary
- 2-3 sprigs peppermint
- 2-3 stalks lemongrass

Method:

1. Take 2 cups of water in a vessel
2. Add all ingredients except green tea in it and allow it to boil
3. Once it starts boiling, add green tea, turn off the flame, cover the vessel with a lid and let it steep for about 2-3 minutes
4. Remove lid, strain into a cup and sip warm

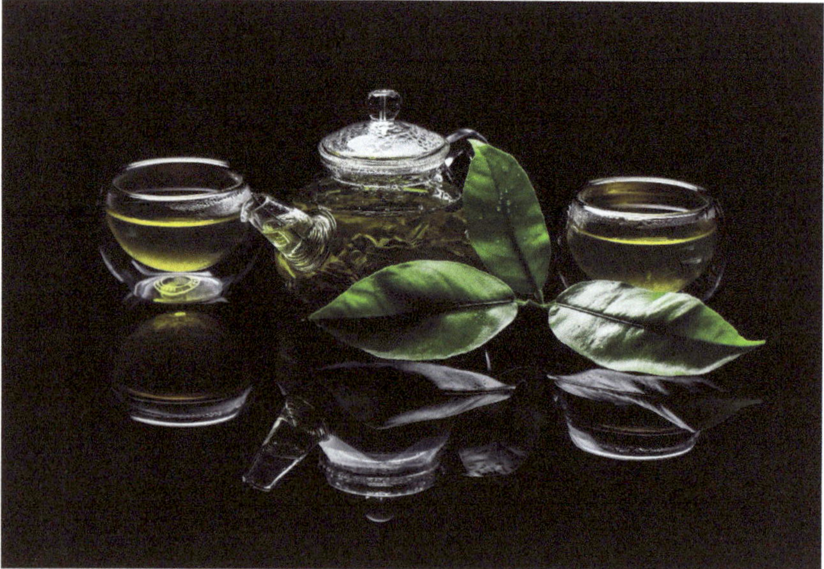

Herbal Tea

Ingredients:

- 1 tbsp chamomile buds
- ¼ tsp oregano
- 1 tsp fennel
- ½ tsp carom
- Pinch of pepper
- 2-3 sprigs thyme
- 1-2 sprigs rosemary
- 2-3 sprigs peppermint
- 2-3 stalks lemongrass
- raw honey/jaggery as per taste

Method:

1. Take 2 cups of water in a vessel
2. Add all ingredients except chamomile in it and allow it to boil
3. Once it starts boiling, add chamomile, turn off the flame, cover the vessel with a lid and let it steep for about 2-3 minutes
4. Remove lid, strain into a cup and sip warm
5. Add raw honey/jaggery to sweeten the beverage

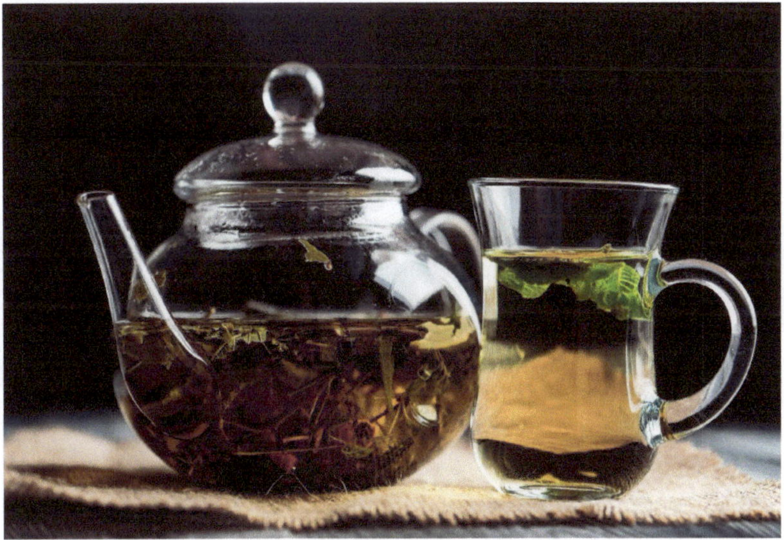

Jal Jeera

Ingredients:

- 3-4 cups water
- 2 1/2 tsp roasted cumin powder
- 1 tsp fennel seed
- 2 tsp lime juice
- 1/2 tbsp grated ginger
- A few mint leaves
- 1/2 tsp black pepper
- Pinch of asafoetida
- Jaggery/honey to taste
- Black salt or rock salt to taste

Method:

1. Combine all the ingredients (except water) into a processor
2. Grind until all blend well
3. Strain with the strainer
4. Add 3-4 cups of water or as required
5. If you like it sweet, then add raw honey or jaggery as required
6. Garnish with mint leaves

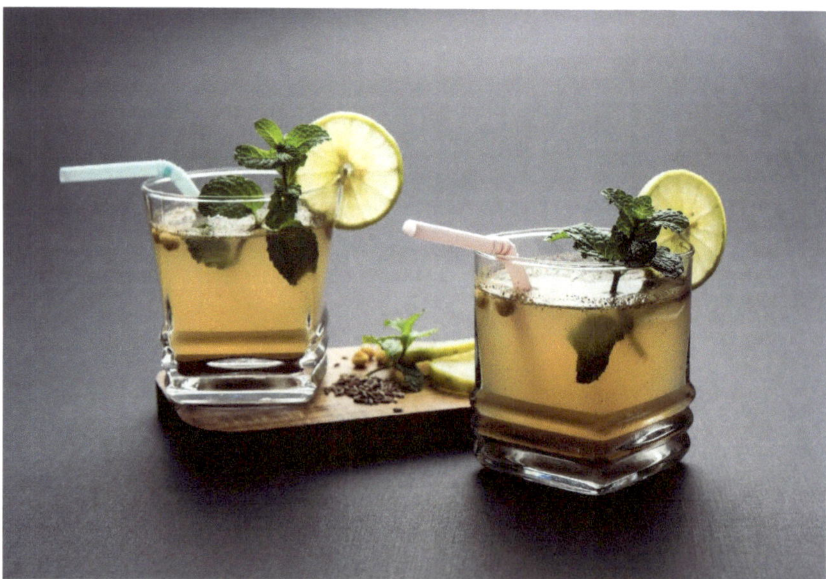

<h1 style="text-align:center">Lemongrass Tea</h1>

Ingredients:

- 2-3 stalks of lemon grass
- 3 to 4 green cardamom
- 1/4 tsp black peppercorns
- 1/4 tsp fennel seeds
- 1 stick of cinnamon
- Few strands of saffron
- A little black tea
- 1/2 tsp fresh grated ginger
- Honey or jaggery as per taste

Method:

1. Boil all of this in 4 cups of water
2. Reduce it to half
3. Add raw honey or jaggery as required

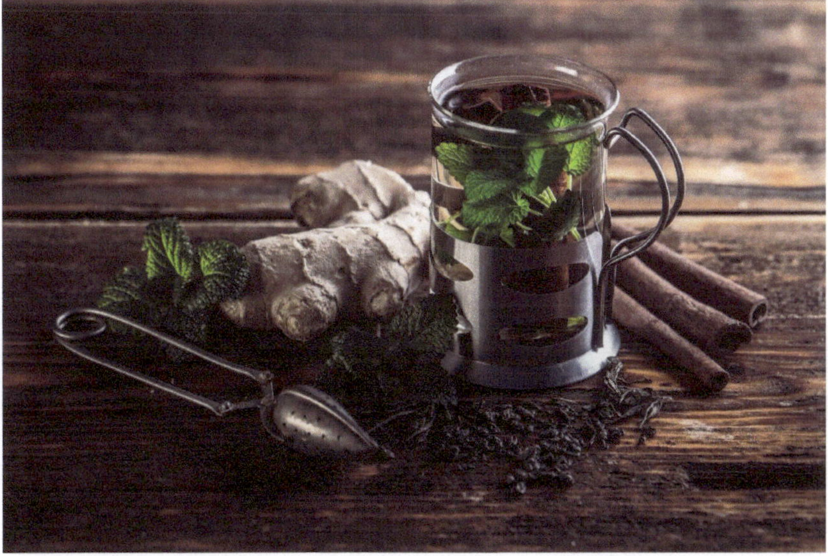

Sattu Buttermilk

Ingredients:

- 2 tbsp sattu powder
- 3 tbsp fresh curd
- 2 cups water
- Pinch of black pepper
- 1/4 tsp roasted cumin powder
- Salt to taste
- 1 tsp lemon juice
- Coriander and mint leaves

Method:

1. Whisk the curd till smooth
2. Add all the ingredients to the curd
3. Dilute with water according to the required consistency
4. Garnish with coriander and mint leaves

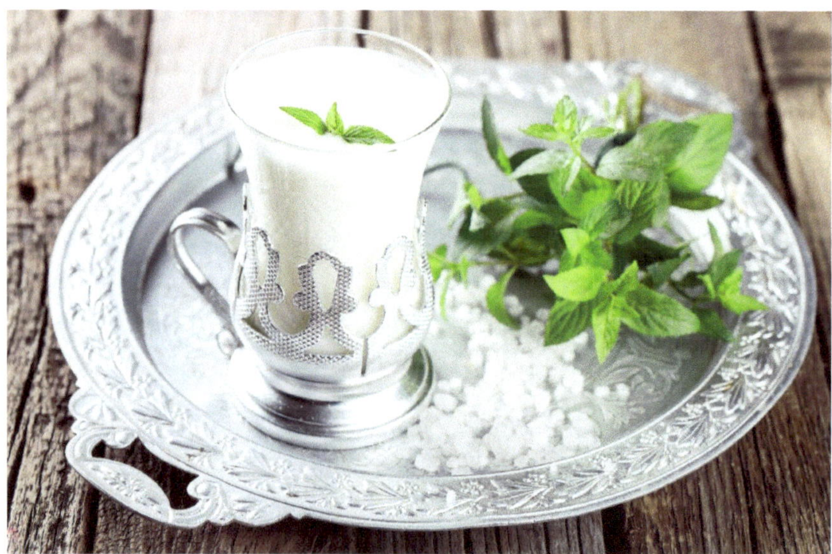

Green Mung Bean Soup

Ingredients:

- ½ cup of green mung
- ½ teaspoon lemon juice
- 1 small green chili
- Small pinch of black pepper
- ½ teaspoon of cumin powder
- A few fresh leaves of mint and coriander for garnishing
- Rock salt or black salt as per taste

Method:

- Wash the green mung thoroughly under running water
- Boil in 4 cups of water until the grains can be properly mashed
- Add lemon, chili, black salt, cumin powder and black pepper powder
- Blend the mixture properly
- Garnish with coriander and mint leaves
- Should be consumed immediately

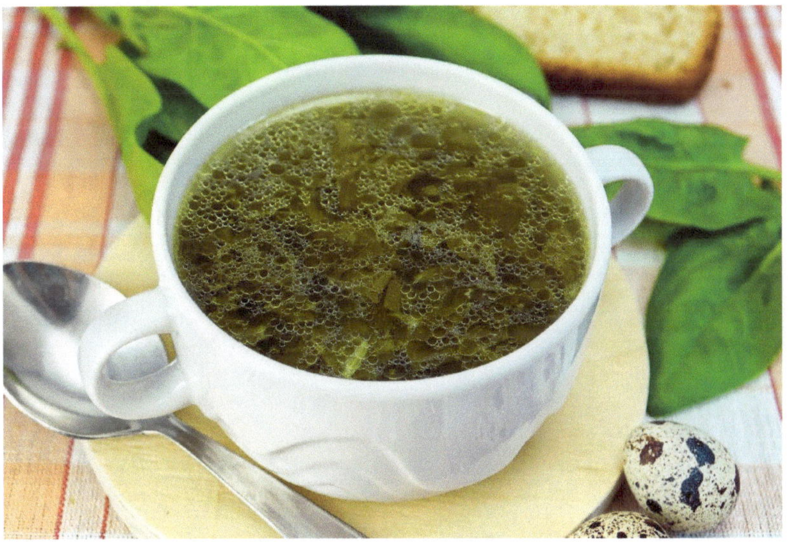

Sattu & Green Peas Soup

Ingredients:

- 1 cup (semi boiled) Green Peas
- 1 tbsp sattu (roasted gram flour)
- 4 cups water
- 1/4 tsp black pepper
- 1/2 tsp cumin powder
- 1/4 tsp ginger- garlic paste
- 1 tsp lime juice
- Pinch of asafoetida
- Salt to taste
- 2 teaspoon pure ghee

Method:

1. Blend the semi-boiled peas into a puree
2. Heat a pan, add ghee and once the ghee heats – add the pureed peas, ginger- garlic paste, asafoetida and sauté
3. Simultaneously, mix sattu flour in 4 cups of water and stir well to avoid lumps
4. Add the sattu mix, pepper powder, salt and cumin powder to the pan and mix well
5. Let it cook on medium flame till the raw smell goes with occasional stirring
6. Just before serving add lime juice

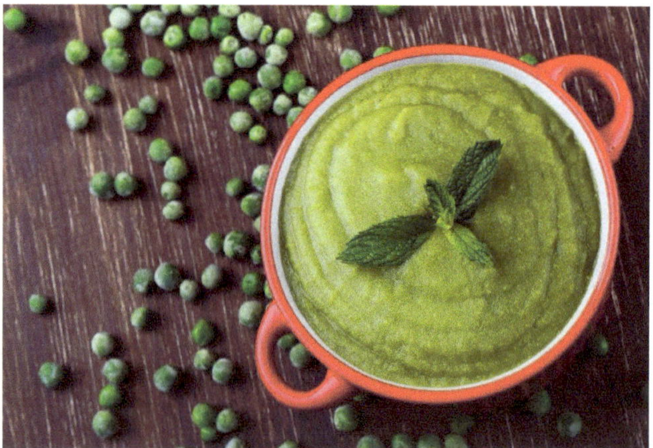

Sweet Potato Soup

Ingredients:

- 500 gm sweet potato
- 1 medium onion
- 2 cloves garlic
- ½ tsp turmeric powder
- Salt and pepper – as per taste
- 3-4 cups water
- 3 sprigs fresh thyme (optional)
- 2 tsp pure ghee
- ½ cup coconut milk (optional)

Method:

1. In a pressure cooker, add ghee over medium-high heat
2. Add onion and garlic and sauté for 5 minutes until tender
3. Add sweet potatoes and sauté for 5 minutes
4. Add salt and pepper as per taste
5. Add water (about 3-4 cups) and boil
6. Cover the pressure cooker and pressure cook for 2 to 3 whistles
7. Using a hand blender, puree the soup in the pot until smooth
8. Add thyme, turmeric, coconut milk and cook for 2-3 mins more
9. Consume immediately

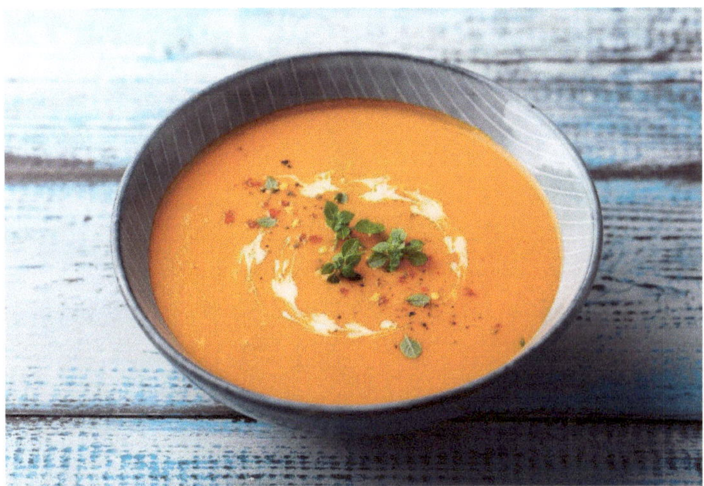

Pumpkin Soup

Ingredients:

- 1 onion
- 2 medium carrots
- 1 handful split peas (pre-soaked)
- 1 cup pumpkin (yellow)
- 1 tbsp fresh ginger garlic paste
- 4 cups water
- Salt, black pepper, red paprika, turmeric, thyme – to taste
- 1 tbsp parsley, chopped
- 1 cup spinach leaves
- 1 tbsp cold pressed coconut oil

Method:

1. Peel and slice onions, slice carrots.
2. Heat a tablespoon of coconut oil in a pot, then add the vegetables and cook on medium, stirring regularly, for a couple of minutes, until the vegetables soften.
3. Then add split peas, pumpkin, ginger garlic paste, spinach and pour over water. Add more water if needed.
4. Add salt, black pepper, red paprika, turmeric, thyme to taste, bring to a boil and then cook on low flame for about 30 minutes, or until the lentils and vegetables are cooked thoroughly.
5. Remove about half the soup from pot and blend it with an immersion blender.
6. Blend until smooth to your liking, then add it back to the rest of the soup and stir to combine.
7. Serve hot.

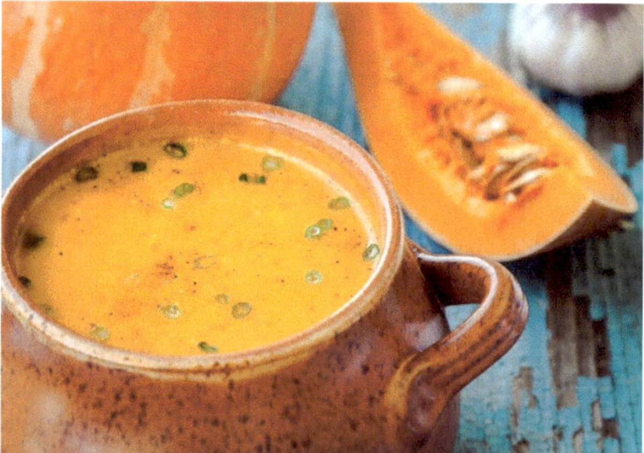

<h1 style="text-align:center">Vegetables Stew</h1>

Ingredients:

- ½ tbsp pure ghee
- 1 tsp garam masala
- ½ onion, sliced
- 5 French beans
- ½ carrot
- ½ potato
- 3 tbsp peas
- 10 florets cauliflower
- 2 green chilies
- 1 cup water
- 1 tsp salt
- 2 cup coconut milk

Instructions:

1. In a large pan, heat ½ tbsp pure ghee
2. Further, add ½ sliced onion and sauté till they shrink slightly. Do not brown the onions.
3. Add beans, carrot, potato, peas, cauliflower, green chilli and 1 tsp garam masala. Sauté for a minute.
4. Add water and salt. Mix well.
5. Cover and boil for 5 minutes or till vegetables are half cooked
6. Now add coconut milk and mix well
7. Boil for 7-8 minutes or till vegetables are cooked completely

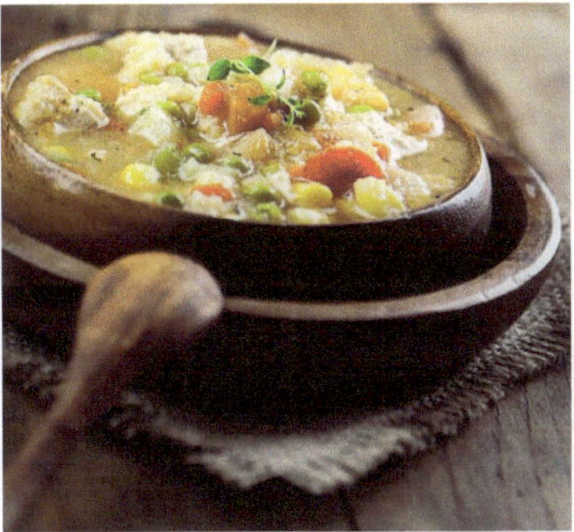

Lentils

Ingredients:

- ½ bowl lentils
- 1 tomato
- 1 onion
- Small piece of ginger
- 1 green chili
- 5-6 cloves of garlic
- ½ teaspoon of garam masala
- ¼ teaspoon turmeric
- Salt and red chili powder as per taste
- Coriander leaves for garnishing

Method:

- Add 2 cups of water, ½ bowl lentils, ¼ teaspoon turmeric powder, salt and red chili according to your taste
- Cook it in a pressure cooker till we get 4 or 5 whistles for a soft and tender consistency
- Add garam masala, tomato cubes, sliced onion, grated ginger, chili and garlic and cook it for another 1-2 whistle
- Garnish with coriander leaves

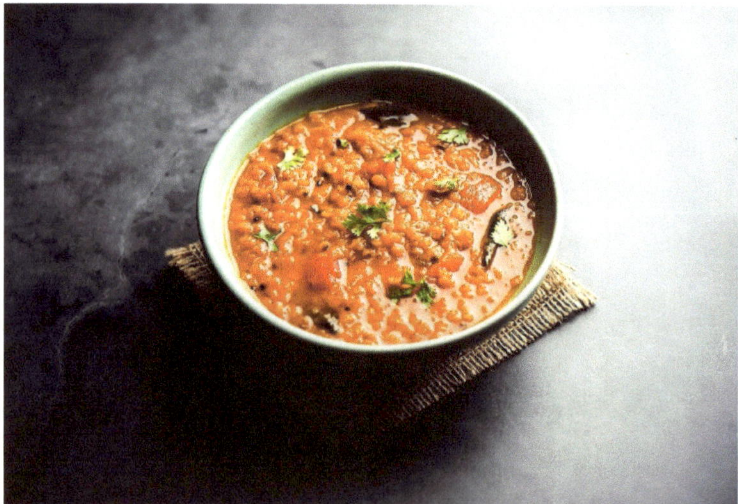

Vegetable Curry

Ingredients:

- ½ bowl vegetable pieces
- 1 tomato
- 1 onion
- Small piece of ginger
- 1 green chili
- 5-6 cloves of garlic
- ½ teaspoon of garam masala
- ¼ teaspoon turmeric
- Salt and red chili powder as per taste
- Coriander leaves for garnishing

Method:

- Cut the seasonal vegetables like carrot, turnip, cauliflower and capsicum in small pieces
- Make a paste of ginger, garlic, green chili and tomatoes
- Boil the vegetables
- Take a pan, put 1 teaspoon of pure ghee/mustard oil, let the cumin seeds and asafoetida splitter
- Add onions and sauté until onion turns golden brown
- Add the tomato paste, garam masala, turmeric, red chili, salt and all the boiled vegetables and cook it for 5 minutes
- Garnish with coriander leaves

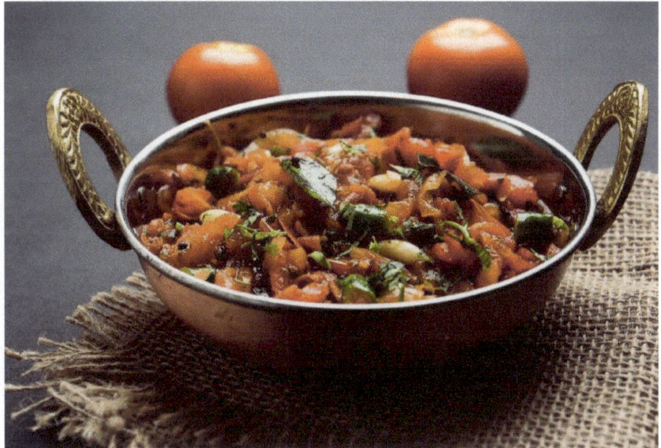

Green Mung Bean khichdi

Ingredients:

- ½ bowl green mung and ½ bowl rice
- ½ teaspoon of garam masala
- 1 teaspoon pure ghee
- Pinch of cumin seeds and asafoetida
- ¼ teaspoon turmeric
- Salt as per taste
- Coriander leaves and Mint leaves
- 1 green chili, a small piece of ginger and 4-5 cloves of garlic
- 1 teaspoon lemon juice

Method:

- Wash green mung and rice and soak it for half an hour
- Pressure cook it with three times of water, turmeric powder and salt till 4 whistles
- Take a pan, put 1 teaspoon of pure ghee, let the cumin seeds and asafoetida splitter
- Add garam masala and boiled mung and rice to the pan
- Mix well and serve in a plate
- Grind some coriander leaves, mint leaves, green chili, small piece of ginger, garlic cloves, lemon juice and salt to make chutney
- Consume khichdi with this delicious chutney

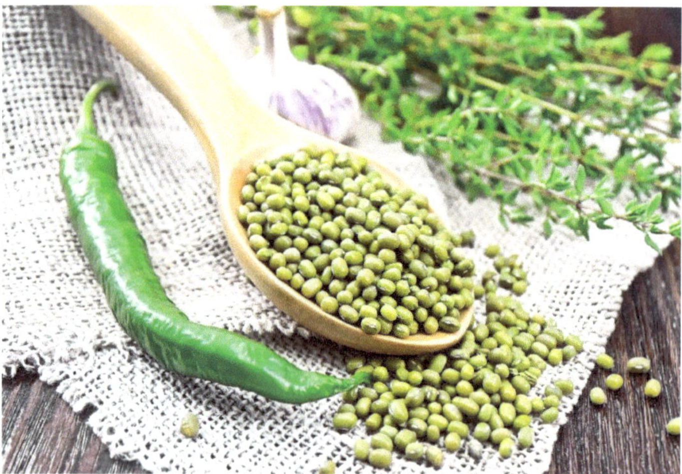

Beetroot Khichdi

Ingredients:

- 4 tbsp rice/brown rice
- 2 tbsp green mung beans
- 1/2 beetroot
- 5-6 cloves of garlic
- Salt to taste
- 1/4 tsp cumin seeds
- 1/4 tsp asafoetida
- 1 tsp pure ghee
- 2 cups water

Instructions:

1. Wash and soak the rice and green mung beans for 2-3 hours
2. Rinse the soaked rice and mung beans with enough water
3. Heat ghee in a pressure cooker and add asafoetida and cumin seeds
4. Once it starts sizzling, add beetroot and crushed or minced garlic
5. Sauté for a minute or two
6. Drain the water from soaked rice and mung and add to the cooker
7. Sauté for a minute and add salt to taste
8. Stir and add 2 cups of water
9. Close the lid of the pressure cooker and cook it for 4-5 whistles

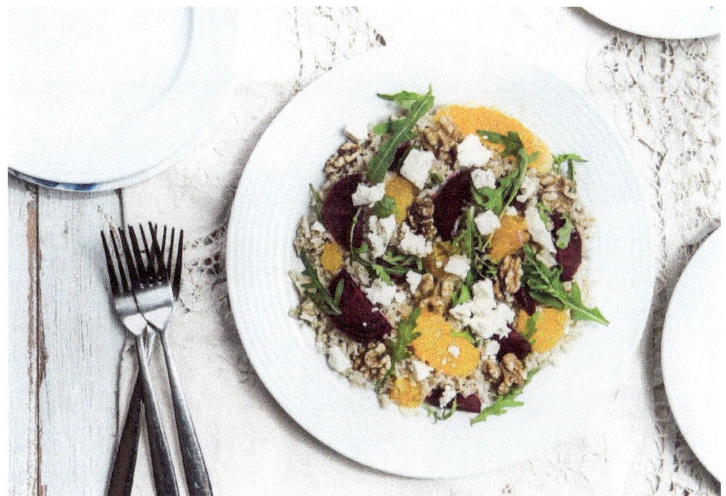

Oats Khichdi

Ingredients:

- ½ bowl yellow mung and ½ bowl oats
- 2 tomatoes
- 1 onion
- 4-5 cloves of garlic
- ½ teaspoon of garam masala
- 1 teaspoon pure ghee
- Pinch of cumin seeds and asafoetida
- ¼ teaspoon turmeric
- Salt as per taste
- Coriander leaves, 1 green chili and grated ginger for garnish

Method:

- Wash mung and soak it for an hour
- Dry roast the oats
- Put pure ghee in a cooker, add some cumin seeds, asafoetida and onions
- Sauté all on medium flame
- Add chopped tomatoes, garlic, yellow mung, oats, turmeric, garam masala and salt
- Pressure cook it with small amount of water till 2-3 whistles (till mung cooks well)
- Garnish with coriander leaves, 1 green chili and grated ginger

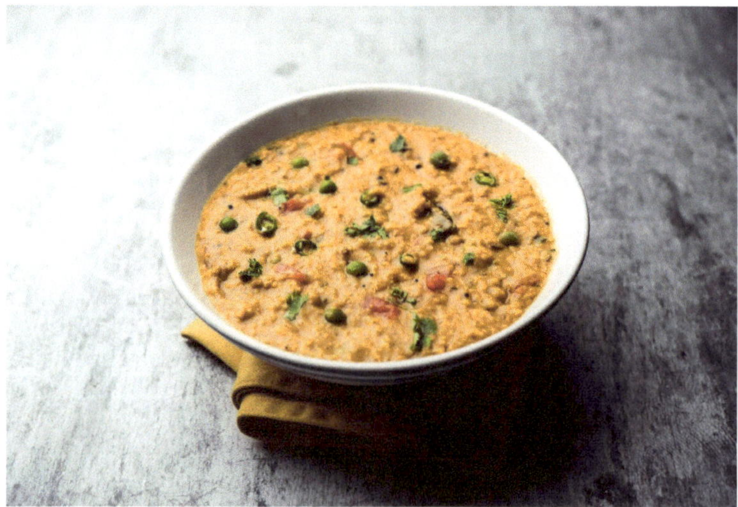

Wheat Daliya

Ingredients:

- ½ bowl yellow mung and ½ bowl roasted wheat daliya
- 1 bowl of mix veggies like carrot, peas, cauliflower, spinach, tomatoes
- 4-5 cloves of garlic
- ½ teaspoon of garam masala
- 1 teaspoon pure ghee
- Pinch of cumin seeds and asafoetida
- ¼ teaspoon turmeric
- Salt as per taste
- Coriander leaves, 1 green chili and grated ginger for garnish

Method:

- Wash mung and soak it for 30 minutes
- Pressure cook daliya and yellow mung by adding 3 times of water till 4 whistles
- Take a pan, put 1 teaspoon of pure ghee, let the cumin seeds and asafoetida splitter
- Add all the vegetables, garlic, garam masala, turmeric, salt and cook properly
- Add boiled daliya and yellow mung
- Garnish with coriander leaves, 1 green chili and grated ginger

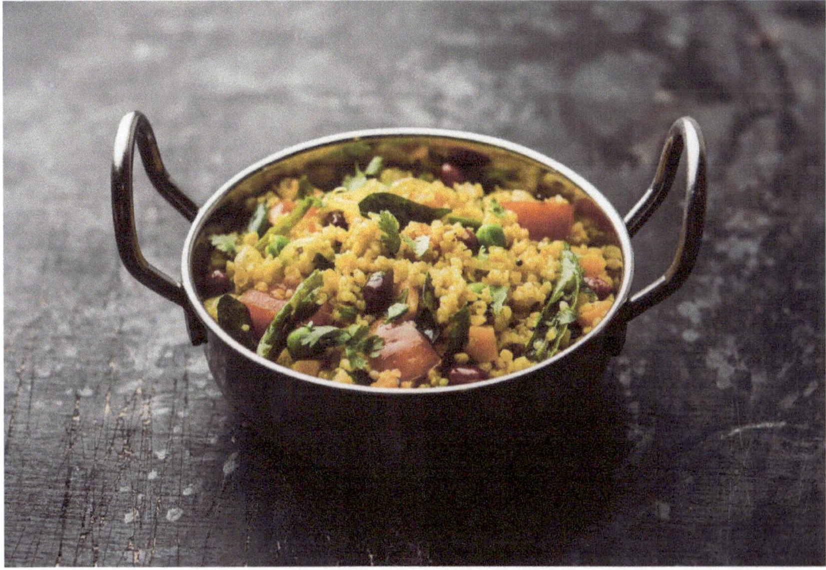

Brown Rice Pulao

Ingredients:

- 1 cup brown rice
- 2 tomatoes, 2 onions, 1 capsicum, 1 carrot, handful of peas
- 1 teaspoon ginger, garlic paste
- ½ teaspoon of garam masala
- 1 teaspoon pure ghee
- Pinch of cumin seeds and asafoetida
- Salt as per taste
- Coriander leaves and 1 green chili for garnish

Method:

- Wash and soak brown rice for minimum 1 hour
- Pressure cook by adding 4 times of water till 1 whistle
- Chop 2 onions, 2 tomatoes, 1 capsicum, 1 carrot and some peas
- Take a pan, put 1 teaspoon of pure ghee, let the cumin seeds and asafoetida splitter
- Add all the vegetables, ginger-garlic paste, garam masala, salt and cook properly
- Add cooked rice as soon as the veggies become crunchy
- Garnish with coriander leaves, 1 green chili and grated ginger

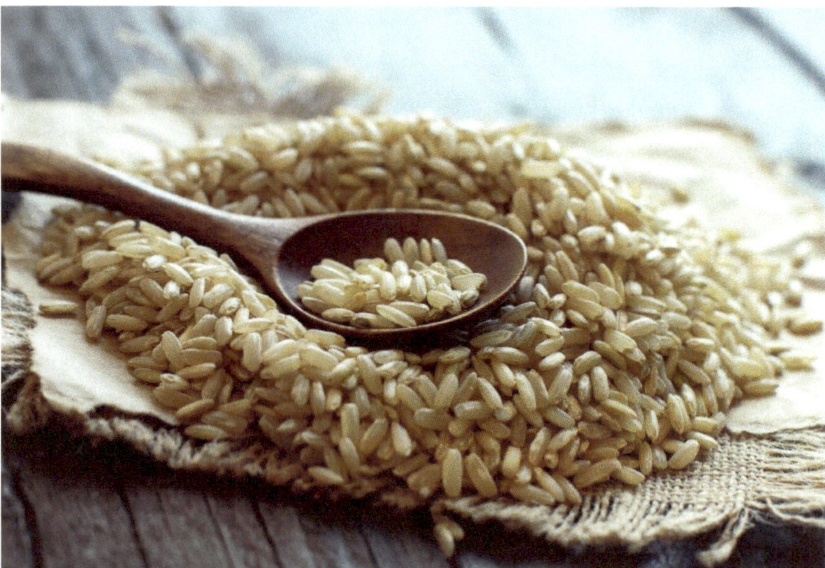

Cashew Dip

Ingredients:

- ¼ cup cashews
- 2-3 cloves garlic
- ½ cup basil leaves
- Few sprigs of parsley/celery for garnishing
- Rock salt to taste

Method:

1. Blend all ingredients into a smooth paste
2. Garnish it with parsley or celery sprigs

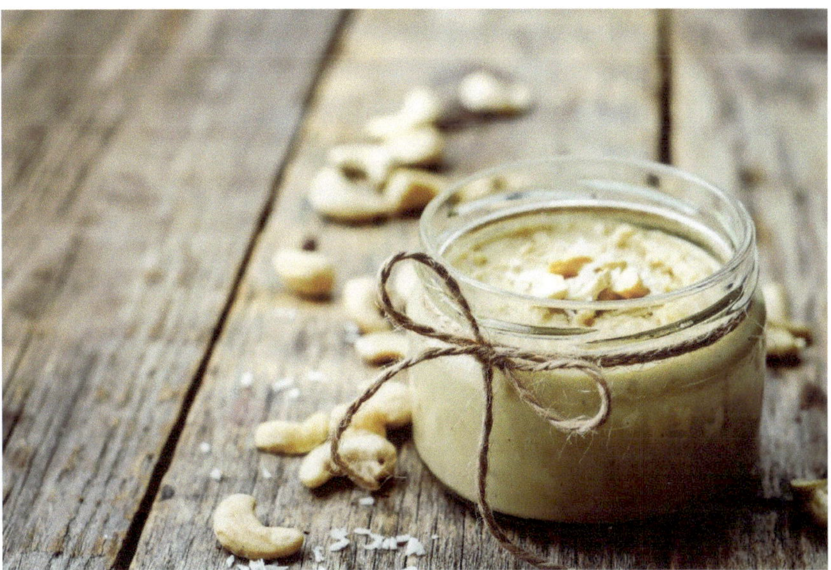

Pea Dip

Ingredients:

- 1 cup peas
- 1/4 cup chopped mint
- 1 lemon
- Rock salt to taste
- Freshly ground pepper

Method:

1. Boil a small pot of water, add the peas and cook for 1 minute
2. Strain and plunge into an ice bath to stop cooking
3. Place blanched peas in a small food processor with mint, lemon zest and juice
4. Puree until smooth
5. Season with salt and pepper
6. Consume immediately

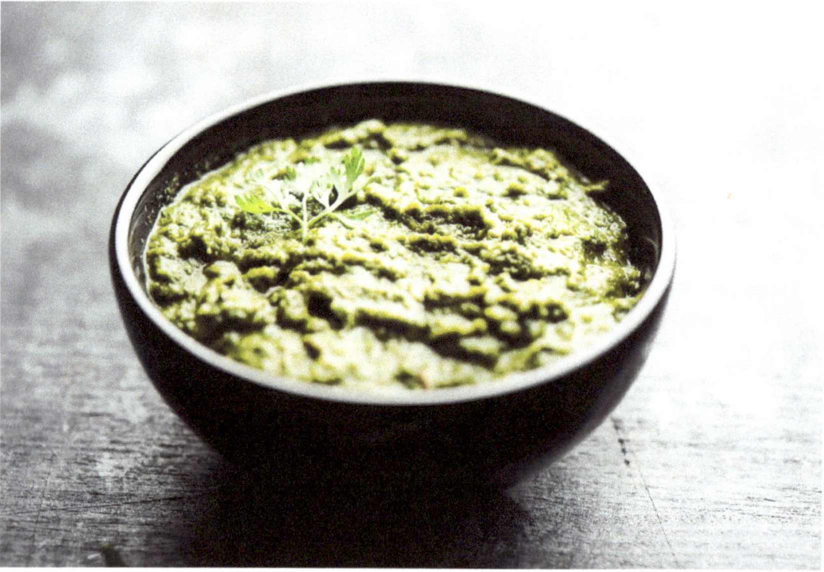

Sweet Potato Hummus

Ingredients:

- 1 large sweet potato
- 1 cup chickpeas
- 1/4 cup water
- 2 tablespoons lemon juice
- 3 tablespoons sesame paste
- 2 cloves garlic
- Salt to taste
- Black pepper to taste

Method:

1. Gather all the ingredients
2. Peel the sweet potato and cut into chunks. Cook in a pot of boiling water for about 10 minutes or until the sweet potato is tender. Mash with a potato masher and set aside to cool.
3. Drain and rinse the chickpeas and add them to a food processor
4. Add the cooled mashed sweet potato, water, freshly squeezed lemon juice, tahini, garlic cloves, salt and pepper
5. Puree until smooth, scraping down the sides with a spatula as needed.
6. Consume with pita or naan bread and sliced vegetables

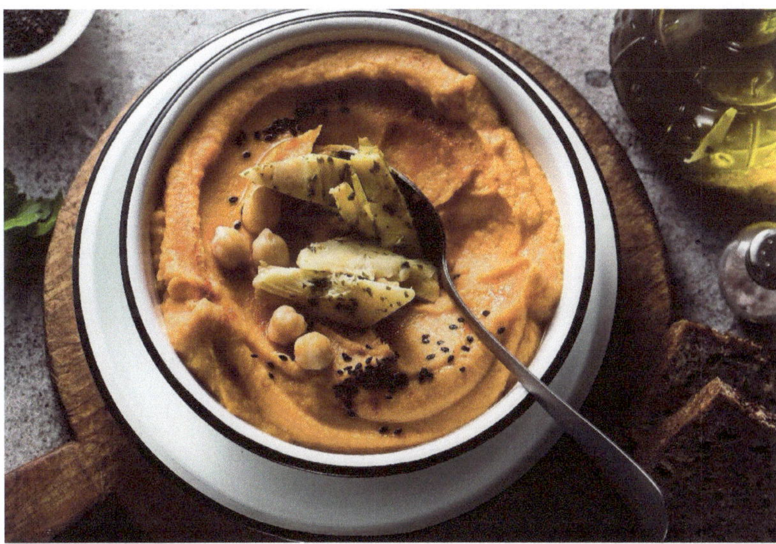

Herbal Dip

Ingredients:

- 1 cup hung curd
- Salt to taste
- ¼ tsp powdered jaggery
- 1tsp lemon juice
- 1 tsp crushed garlic
- 2 tsp olive oil
- 1 tsp black pepper
- 1 tsp mixed herbs

Method:

1. To prepare hung curd – Take an empty bowl and place the strainer on top. Double a kitchen cloth and put it on the strainer. Pour the curd in the cloth, hold up the ends of the cloth and squeeze it gently. Once the water starts draining out, keep it back on the strainer and refrigerate this for 6-8 hours.
2. Take 2 tablespoons of hung curd in a bowl and then add the powdered jaggery to it
3. Add salt according to taste
4. Add crushed garlic and olive oil
5. Add crushed pepper and mixed herbs according to taste
6. Mix well

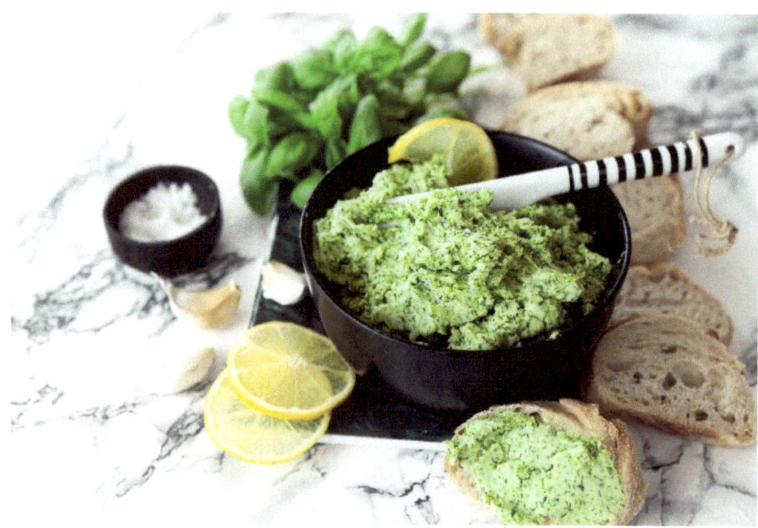

This is it!!

Please note recipes mentioned in this book are general recipes and can easily be modified by replacing the main content. Like, banana salad can be prepared using the recipe of mango salad just by replacing mango with banana. Similarly, any vegetable curry can be prepared by using curry recipe of this book.

These lifestyle and dietary changes give multi-dimensional health benefits.

Set following intentions just after you wake up –

- ➢ I will exercise and walk
- ➢ I will eat good food
- ➢ I will follow the changes mentioned in this book in any circumstances

"Health is Wealth" – They Say!!